Reflexology

Learn How to Use Reflexology With Easy Techniques and Simple Instruction

By Tatyana Williams

Published in Canada

© Copyright 2015 – Tatyana Williams

ISBN-13: 978-1508676348
ISBN-10: 1508676348

Table of Contents

Introduction 1

Understanding Reflexology.............................1

Chapter 1: Reflexology Basics 5

Chapter 2: Getting Started 9

Chapter 3: The Foot Reflexology 13

Chart Map...13

The Hand Reflexology....................................15

Chart Map...15

The Ear Reflexology 16

Chart Map...16

Chapter 4: Self-Practice With 17

Foot Reflexology 17

Chapter 5: Self-Practice With 21

Hand Reflexology..21

Chapter 6: Self-Practice With 23

Ear Reflexology 23

Chapter 7: Five DIY Reflexology Techniques by

Ailment...25

Chapter 8: Hand Reflexology: 37

Specific Tips & Techniques 37

Chapter 9: Foot Reflexology: Specific Tips &

Techniques..39

Chapter 10: Ear Reflexology:.....................41

Specific Tips & Techniques 41

Conclusion..43

Introduction
Understanding Reflexology

What can reflexology do?

Reflexology can be used to help relieve physical pain and reduce psychological components of illnesses, such as depression and anxiety.

What can reflexology not do?

Treat or cure any illness. Reflexology is not the cure for cancer – or even the common cold. However, just as cold remedies are used to treat the symptoms of a cold, so reflexology can be used to alleviate the symptoms of certain ailments.

While it is not known to cure or treat any illness, reflexology is recognized by the Mayo clinic as a method of pain relief and reduction of stress relief for people with a variety of ailments and illnesses. The practice has been as an alternative method of symptom treatment since the time of the ancient Egyptians. There are many professional reflexologists, but reflexology is also a technique that you can do at home.

Before you can start practicing reflexology at home, however, you need to have a basic understanding of what it is and how can be used for pain and psychological symptom relief.

So, what exactly is the practice of reflexology?

When referring to reflexology people are talking about the process of applying pressure to specific areas of the hands and feet or even the ear. In essence, it is a form of therapeutic massage, based on the theory that there are pathways from the hands, feet and ears to other parts of our body, through which we can direct positive, healing energy.

Neither lotion nor oil is used in the practice and the ways by which the pressure is applied depends upon the area you is trying to address. The idea is that certain areas of the ears, feet and hands, known as reflex points, correspond to organs and limbs on the body. Massaging the correct spots on the ear, foot or hand in the right way is believed to relieve pain in those matching areas of the body.

This pressure massage is generally accomplished with the use of fingers, thumbs, and palms, but may also be applied by stepping, pressing or rolling the hands and feet against stones or beads. Beaded foot massagers work on this principle. For reflexology of the hand a small ball such as a golf ball may be used similarly to great effect.

Some of these spots are well known and you may have even used a form of reflexology without knowing that's what you are doing. One popular home remedy for relief of a tooth pain is to massage the area between your thumb and your forefinger. This method works on the same premise as reflexology, though the reflex points for teeth and sinuses are believed to be in a different area of the hand, according to modern reflexology charts.

Reflexology can be an effect, simple treatment to help alleviate symptoms for many people. However, there are people for whom reflexology is not recommended and can be dangerous. If you fall into any of these categories, do not attempt the methods outlined in this book or seek treatment from a reflexologist:

- Women experiencing an unstable pregnancy
- People suffering from deep vein thrombosis or thrombophlebitis
- Anyone with a fever and severe infection
- Someone who has cellulite of the feet or hands
- Anyone who has recently suffered a stroke
- People with cuts, bruises, swelling, inflammation or blisters on the hands, feet or ears
- Other people who should contact a doctor before considering reflexology - and should only have it done by a professional - include:

- Women in their first trimester of pregnancy
- Anyone taking an anti-coagulant drug
- People suffering from cancer
- Diabetics who require insulin
- Anyone with a contagious condition
- Someone who suffers from chronic fatigue, fibromyalgia or other illness that causes extreme sensitivity
- Anyone with epilepsy
- People who have undergone heart surgery recently

Chapter 1:
Reflexology Basics

Consult the Chart

In order for reflexology to be effective, you must first learn the areas of the hands, feet and ears that correspond to the appropriate areas of the body that you want to target. Included later in the book are three reference charts for that purpose. If you only have one or two areas that require pain relief, then you can learn only those areas for now and focus on learning others if different illnesses arise.

When looking over the charts, you will notice that the zones for hands and feet are very similar. If you align big toes and thumbs, and wrists to heels, you will find that the zones line up almost identically, with a few exceptions. For example, the spinal zone on the hand runs from the middle of the inside edge of the thumb down to just below where the wrist begins. On the foot, the same zone is located on the inside edge of the foot, starting in the middle of the big toe and extending down to the middle of the side of the heel. What this means is that, if you have memorized the location of a zone on the foot chart, you should be able to easily locate the corresponding zone on the hand, as well – or vice versa.

Learn the moves

You also need to know the basic techniques for how to massage each area. In some cases, this requires simple, repeated pressure. Sometimes, a rotation of the massaging finger is what is needed. Another technique, known as thumb walking, requires using either of the thumbs to "step' up and down across an area, by pressing down and back up.

Thumb walking is generally used most areas of the feet and the larger zones of the hand. A pressing with rotation is generally most effective on the fingers, toes and palms of the hand, while certain small reflex points, such as just under the ball of the foot, are best activated using direct, repeated, firm pressure for a count of 15-20 seconds. As with any massage, what feels best will generally be the most effective. If it feels like you are relieving the soreness of a muscle, you are likely to be doing it the correct way. If you try one way and it doesn't feel right, try another method and see if that feels better to you.

What are the tools of the trade?

As stated earlier, typically the only tools needed are the fingers, thumbs and palms, but other implements may be used as well. Smooth stones, small balls, beaded rollers and pebbled pathways can all be used to bring about the effects of reflexology. These may be especially helpful for those who wish to perform DIY reflexology, but lack the mobility to reach their own feet with their hands. These are also helpful for people who may lack grip strength in their hands, since they can use the ball to apply the pressure, rather than their own finger and thumb power.

In lieu of oil or lotion, talcum powder or cornstarch may be used to help assist with movement and to combat moisture from sweat.

What to expect when you're reflexing

Depending on how long and intense the session is, how much tension has been built up in the area or just how your particular body is wired, you may expect to have a host of possible reactions during and after your reflexology session.

These reactions include, but are not limited to:

- Laughing
- Crying
- Fatigue
- Increased thirst
- Flatulence
- Feeling cold
- Feeling light-headed
- Sweating
- Coughing
- Sighing
- Belching
- Minor muscle spasms

Chapter 2:
Getting Started

Now that you know the basics, it's time to get ready for your first DIY reflexology session. Whether you are performing reflexology on yourself or a friend, it is important to prepare the area in advance, particularly if you are just beginning to try the techniques. You want to pick the right room and environment for the reflexology session, as well as making sure your tools are readily at hand when you need them. You also need to make sure that you are relaxed, even if you are performing the techniques on someone else.

The area for the session should be cool and quiet. You want to have an atmosphere in the room that promotes relaxation, so low lighting might also be helpful. Scented candles or incense and soft, soothing music are not necessary, but they might make the room more peaceful and conducive to healing.

If you are massaging your own reflexes, make sure that you have a comfortable place to sit or lie down. Sitting up is recommended if you cannot reach your feet. In this way you can roll your foot around on a ball without risk of falling down. If you are massaging someone else, make sure they have a comfortable place to sit or lie down and that you have a comfortable, easily moved place to sit while you massage their hands, ears, and feet.

Gather your charts, talcum powder and any tools you may be using and keep them close at hand. Before you start on yourself, you should take a self-assessment. To do this, make a list of any and all illnesses and complaints you've been having problems with recently such as heartburn, headaches, insomnia, pain, etc. You should number these in order of importance, so that you can start with the worst ailment and work your way down to the least problematic symptom. Refer to your charts as needed to make sure you are targeting all the correct areas.

If you are performing the treatment on another person, stop and ask them specific questions about where their physical complaints are. You may want to write down their answers, so you can concentrate on all the areas of suffering. As with your own list, have them number the complaints in order of importance.

Before starting the session *make sure they do not fit the categories mentioned earlier for people who should not receive reflexology*. Serious complications can arise for those categories of people, if they use reflexology. The last thing you want is for your friend to end up in the hospital because you released a blood clot from their foot.

Whether you are self-practicing or performing the techniques on another person, before you begin, you should take a moment to calm yourself before beginning. Start by sitting in a comfortable position in your seat. Close your eyes and take several slow, deep breaths, in through your nose and out through your mouth. If you are helping someone else, have them do the same.

Chapter 3:
The Foot Reflexology
Chart Map

This chart outlines the main reflex point zones of the foot. Not all charts are exactly the same, as some will have fewer or more zones, but these are the basic zones and are a good starting place for beginners who are just learning the art of reflexology.

Foot Reflexology Chart

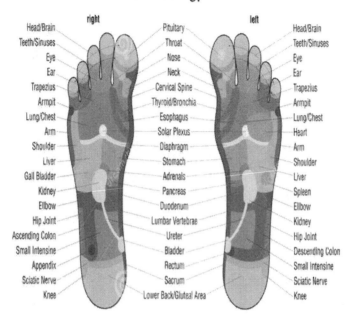

right

Head/Brain
Teeth/Sinuses
Eye
Ear
Trapezius
Armpit
Lung/Chest
Arm
Shoulder
Liver
Gall Bladder
Kidney
Elbow
Hip Joint
Ascending Colon
Small Intensine
Appendix
Sciatic Nerve
Knee

Pituitary
Throat
Nose
Neck
Cervical Spine
Thyroid/Bronchia
Esophagus
Solar Plexus
Diaphragm
Stomach
Adrenals
Pancreas
Duodenum
Lumbar Vertebrae
Ureter
Bladder
Rectum
Sacrum
Lower Back/Gluteal Area

left

Head/Brain
Teeth/Sinuses
Eye
Ear
Trapezius
Armpit
Lung/Chest
Heart
Arm
Shoulder
Liver
Spleen
Elbow
Kidney
Hip Joint
Descending Colon
Small Intensine
Sciatic Nerve
Knee

The Hand Reflexology Chart Map

Hand Reflexology Chart

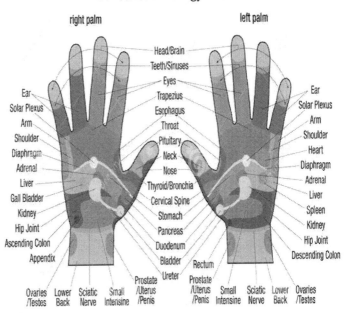

right palm | left palm

Head/Brain
Teeth/Sinuses
Eyes
Trapezius
Esophagus
Throat
Pituitary
Neck
Nose
Thyroid/Bronchia
Cervical Spine
Stomach
Pancreas
Duodenum
Bladder
Ureter

Ear
Solar Plexus
Arm
Shoulder
Diaphragm
Adrenal
Liver
Gall Bladder
Kidney
Hip Joint
Ascending Colon
Appendix

Ear
Solar Plexus
Arm
Shoulder
Heart
Diaphragm
Adrenal
Liver
Spleen
Kidney
Hip Joint
Descending Colon

Rectum

Prostate /Uterus /Penis

Ovaries /Testes | Lower Back | Sciatic Nerve | Small Intensine | Prostate /Uterus /Penis | Prostate /Uterus /Penis | Small Intensine | Sciatic Nerve | Lower Back | Ovaries /Testes

The Ear Reflexology Chart Map

Ear Reflexology Chart

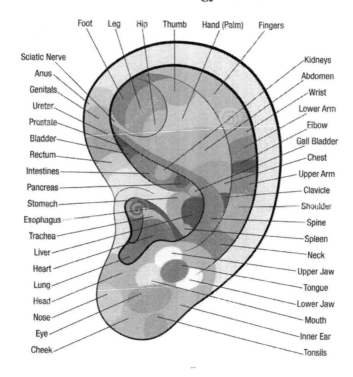

Foot · Leg · Hip · Thumb · Hand (Palm) · Fingers

Sciatic Nerve
Anus
Genitals
Ureter
Prostate
Bladder
Rectum
Intestines
Pancreas
Stomach
Esophagus
Trachea
Liver
Heart
Lung
Head
Nose
Eye
Cheek

Kidneys
Abdomen
Wrist
Lower Arm
Elbow
Gall Bladder
Chest
Upper Arm
Clavicle
Shoulder
Spine
Spleen
Neck
Upper Jaw
Tongue
Lower Jaw
Mouth
Inner Ear
Tonsils

Chapter 4:
Self-Practice With
Foot Reflexology

Follow all the steps listed under Getting Started to prepare yourself for the session, including selecting a comfortable area, making and rating a list of ailments, and gathering your tools and charts. Take a few moments to relax yourself via deep breaths before you begin.

If at any time during the session you begin to tense up or feel stressed, stop and take a moment to relax again. Close your eyes and breathe slowly in through your nose and out through your mouth a few times, until the tension drains out of your muscles.

If you are able to pull your foot into your lap, then you will follow the methods outlined for using the thumbs and fingers to massage the reflexes. If you are *not*

able to pull your foot into your lap, or if you simply lack
the appropriate strength in your hands to apply adequate
pressure, then use the methods for the ball massage
technique.

When practicing foot reflexology on yourself, it is
best to be in a seated position. Foot reflexology can be
done from a chair, a couch or on the side of the bed (as
long as your feet reach the floor, if you are using the ball
method).

Thumb and finger massage

Concentrating on the areas you located during your
self-assessment, begin with the most problematic area.
Referring to your chart if necessary, find the appropriate
area of the foot. Using the thumb walking method, rock
your thumb into the problem area, pressing firmly, but
not so hard as to cause discomfort. Walk across the
whole zone at least twice, spending up to 2 minutes for
the worst or larger areas, or about 30 seconds for smaller
zones and lesser ailments. In zones where pressure is
needed instead of thumb walking, press firmly into the
area for about 20 seconds. Release and repeat twice more.
If the pain is bilateral or the zone is present on both feet,
repeat on the other foot.

Ball massage

Place a ball 1-1.5" in diameter on the floor in front of your chair. Raise your foot above the ball and lower it so that the correct zone is on the ball. Firmly step down with your foot and roll, rock or press the ball against the area until the entire zone has been massaged, spending 2 minutes for the worst areas and 30 seconds for smaller ones. When apply pressure only, press and hold for 20 seconds, release and repeat twice. Repeat on the other foot as needed.

Chapter 5:
Self-Practice With
Hand Reflexology

This is a simple method that can be performed at any time, without the need to prepare in advance. Whether you are at work or in the car or at the theater or somewhere else, you can still give yourself this simple massage and help alleviate sudden pains and problems that might arise when you are not able to have a full session. This technique can be done while sitting or while lying down. In the bath is an excellent place to perform this type of self-reflexology.

Of course, in order to do this method in public, you need to either memorize the chart map or keep a small copy on your person. It might be simplest to memorize only those areas that you are likely to need while away from home, such as the reflex point for the head and neck, if you are prone to getting headaches.

As with self-practice foot reflexology, hand reflexology can be practiced with the thumb and fingers of the other hand or through use of a small ball. Either way, the instructions will be basically the same.

Find the area on the chart that matches where the pain is. Using your thumb, finger or a ball, apply rotating pressure in the spot that corresponds to the right area of the body. This should take 10-20 seconds, depending on the size of the zone. Repeat on the other hand, as necessary. On areas such as the base of the thumb where direct pressure is not ideal, thumb walk or rock the ball over the zone from one side to the other.

Chapter 6:
Self-Practice With
Ear Reflexology

This is perhaps the easiest method of DIY reflexology. As with hand reflexology, it can be done anywhere, with relative privacy and ease, though if you do not wish to take a holistic approach and work the entire ear, that will require learning the zones or keeping a chart on your person.

You can perform this technique sitting up or lying down. It can be done in the bath, but special care should be taken not to get water into your ears.

Using the finger and thumb of one hand, massage the area of the ear that corresponds to the problem area on the map. Use a firm rolling motion. Use pressure, but do not pinch. Roll the area between your thumb and finger – or with just your finger on the attached areas of the ear – for a count of 10. Repeat as necessary until you have received relief or until you have massaged for one minute, whichever comes first. Repeat on the other ear, if the pain is bilateral.

Chapter 7:
Five DIY Reflexology
Techniques by Ailment

What follows are some simple shortcuts for combating a few common ailments, through the use of self-directed reflexology. When you are unclear on where the zone or reflex point described is located, please refer to the chart images for clarification.

1. Relieving lower back pain and sciatica

As we age, lower back problem can become a frequent problem for many of us, particularly if we have sustained an injury to the lower back in the past. And when the sciatic nerve is involved, the pain may extend down into one or both hips.

Back treatment can be costly and time consuming. When the pain is not acute, often times we will just suffer through it without doing much to relieve the symptoms other than taking over the counter pain relief.

Reflexology provides an alternative method to try and combat the pain and muscle spasms of the lower back and sciatic nerve area.

Foot Method

The zones relating to the lower back and the sciatic nerve are located on the lower half of the heel and the line delineating the middle of the heel, respectively. If you are self-practicing, use the ball method to roll over this area, from the outside of the foot to the inside, twice to three times per foot, on both feet. Alternatively, have someone else thumb walk all the way across the lower back zone of the heel, from outside to inside, twice to three times per foot, on both feet. Repeat on the line for the sciatic nerve. If the pain is not lessened, repeat a second time.

Hand Method

The zones correlating to the lower back and sciatic nerve are actually on the wrist, rather than on the hand itself. The sciatic nerve zone is the outline of the bottom of the palm where hand meets wrist and the lower back zone is the whole area that extends an inch or so below that – excluding a small circular area on either side, just below the palm.

Ear Method

There is no reflex point zone on the ear relating to the lower back, but the spinal zone is just outside the opening to the ear canal. The sciatic nerve zone is located in a very small area just next to the front curve of the ear. Take a straight pin with a ball head on it – press an eraser onto the sharp point of the pin for safety - and press the ball into the areas, using a rocking motion for the spine zone and rotating firmly for several seconds in the sciatic nerve zone. Repeat on the other ear, if the pain is bilateral.

2. Relieving tension and stress

Tension builds up in our bodies when we are stressed out or worried about things. This translates into tight muscles and can lead to headaches and other problems. The reason this happens is because our brain transmits signals via our nerves, triggering defense mechanisms that cause our shoulders and other body parts to hunch and tighten up, in preparation for a fight or flight response. Therefore, in order to combat tension, we should go after the nerve centers of our bodies, which are located in the brain and the spine. Working the reflex points for these areas may also help to alleviate the pain from a headache.

Foot Method

The reflex point zone for the spine starts on the middle of the outside edge of the big toe of each foot and extends downward to the outside edge of the middle of the heel. The toe end corresponds to the cervical spine and so on, with the edge of the heel representing the sacrum. The zone for the brain and head goes across the top of each toe where the pad is, except the big toe, where it extends about halfway down the pad of the toe.

Using your thumbs or a ball, apply a rotating pressure to the top of each toe, one at a time on both feet. Start with the big toe and work your way outward. Then either thumb walk or roll the ball along the inside edge of the foot starting mid-big toe and continuing downward to middle of the heel. Repeat on the other foot. Do this one or three times, as needed to reduce tension.

Hand Method

The reflex point zone on the hand which is related to the spine runs from the middle of the outside edge of the thumb down to just below where the wrist begins. The zone for the head is on the pads of all four fingers and the top half of the pad for the thumb.

Using rotating pressure with a finger or thumb, massage each finger tip separately, beginning with the thumb and working your way outward to the pinkie finger. Repeat on the other hand. Next, thumb walk down from the middle of the outside edge of the thumb, down to just under the palm on the wrist. Repeat on the other hand. Do this one to three times until tension subsides.

Ear Method

On the ear the spinal zone is located just outside the opening to the ear canal. The brain zone is near the top of earlobe, on the side closest to head. Rock along the spinal zone of each ear, using the ball head of a straight pin – sharp end capped with an eraser for safety. Gently but firmly massage the reflex point for the brain between your thumb and forefinger.

3. Fighting fatigue and increasing energy and alertness

There are any number of reasons why you may be tired and not feeling as alert as you need to be. Perhaps you did not get a good night's sleep before work, maybe your children have exhausted you, but it is several hours before they can be sent to bed, or maybe you are making a long road trip. Either way, fatigue can be anything from inconvenient to dangerous.

Using reflexology may help combat fatigue by targeting various glands that regulate energy and areas of the body related to breathing so that we can get more oxygen which helps us be more alert. The adrenal glands and thyroid gland are responsible for combating fatigue and helping stay mentally alert. The solar plexus and the diaphragm help regulate our breathing and make us feel more centered and focused in our energy.

Foot Method

The reflex points for the adrenal glands are located almost directly in the center of the foot. The thyroid reflex point is located in a diagonal that runs from the split of the first two toes toward the outside of the foot where the base of the big toe connects. The reflex point zones for the solar plexus and diaphragm are located under the ball of the foot. The solar plexus zone is almost directly in the middle of this line, straight down from the second toe, while the diaphragm zone makes up the line that runs underneath the ball.

Using your finger, thumb or the ball method, apply direct pressure to the center point of the foot for 20 seconds, then release and repeat two more times. Do this on both feet. Next, using your finger, thumb or a ball, move along the line of the thyroid zone in a walking or rotating motion, starting on the outside of the foot and working inward. Do this a couple of times. Repeat on the other foot.

Next, press your finger into the area for the solar plexus and press upward for 20 seconds. Release and repeat twice. Thumb walk across the bottom outline of the ball of the foot, from the outside to the inside. Do this twice. Repeat both processes on the other foot.

Hand Method

The reflex points for the adrenal glands are located almost directly in the center of the hand. The thyroid reflex point is located across the bottom knuckle of the thumb, just above the fleshy part of the palm. The solar plexus reflex point is located just below the pad for the middle finger. The diaphragm runs along the outline for the padding of the first three fingers.

Using your finger, apply direct pressure with a mild rotation to the center of the palm. Do this for 20 seconds, then release. Repeat twice more. Do the whole process again on the other hand. Using the thumb of the other hand, thumb walk around the bottom knuckle of your thumb from the outside and working in. Do this twice. Repeat on the other hand.

Press a finger into the palm, rotating slightly, just underneath the pad of the middle finger. Maintain the rotating pressure for 20 seconds. Repeat twice, then thumb walk across the line for the diaphragm. Repeat both processes on the other hand.

Ear Method

There are no corresponding zones on the ears for these areas.

4. Improving depression

To target depression with reflexology, we want to approach the reflex point zones for the pituitary gland and the hypothalamus, which regulate mood, and those areas of the body which are related to breathing, so that we can get more oxygen, a natural releaser of endorphins. The stimulation of the solar plexus and the diaphragm reflex points can also help make us feel more centered and focused in our energy.

Foot Method

The zone that corresponds to the pituitary gland and hypothalamus is located dead center in the middle of the pad of each big toe. The reflex point zones for the solar plexus and diaphragm are located under the ball of the foot. The solar plexus zone is almost directly in the middle of this line, while the diaphragm zone makes up the line that runs underneath the ball.

Press your thumb into the reflex point for the pituitary gland and use rotating pressure to massage the zone. Do this for about 20 seconds. Release the pressure, then repeat twice more. Repeat on the other foot.

Next, press your finger into the area for the solar plexus and press upward for 20 seconds. Release and repeat twice. Thumb walk across the bottom outline of the ball of the foot, from the outside to the inside. Do this twice. Repeat both processes on the other foot.

Hand Method

Press your thumb into the reflex point for the pituitary gland located on the thumb and use a firm, rotating pressure to massage the zone. Do this for about 20 seconds. Release the pressure, then repeat twice more. Repeat on the other hand.

Press a finger into the palm, rotating slightly, just underneath the pad of the middle finger. Maintain the rotating pressure for 20 seconds. Repeat twice, then thumb walk across the line for the diaphragm. Repeat both processes on the other hand.

Ear Method

There are no corresponding zones on the ears for those areas of the body.

5. Fighting insomnia

There are many reasons for insomnia. If you don't know the reason for your inability to sleep, the best way to attack the problem is to massage all the zones, rather than try to focus on one. This is in order to bring relaxation to all areas and give you a better chance of falling asleep.

If you happen to know the cause of your insomnia, such as stress or stomach upset, you can target those areas of the hands, feet and ears and address the concern directly. Otherwise, follow the suggestions outlined below to target all areas of the body and bring about relaxation.

The foot massage will work best if you can get a partner to help you, but if not, try using the hand or ear method – or try doing the foot massage while in the bath. The warm water "tricks" your brain into thinking the fingers and thumbs are not your own and makes the massage more effective.

Foot Method

Starting with the big toe, massage the pad of each toe in gentle circles, moving down until you have massaged the whole toe. Move from the big to toward the outside of the foot in this way, until you have massaged the pinkie toe. From there, thumb walk down the outside of the pinkie toe and down along the outer edge of the foot, including the padded portion.

Move down the outside of the foot until you reach the heel. Massage the entire heel from the outer edge to the inner edge of the foot. Then thumb walk your way up the inner edge of the foot until you have reached the base of the big toe again.

Work across the ball of your foot, paying attention to each zone within it, until you reach the area that you've already massaged. Now work across and down until you have stimulated every reflex point located in the arch of your foot.

Stop and take a moment to repeat your deep breathing exercises, then repeat this process on the other foot.

Hand Method

Beginning with the thumb, massage the length of each finger with the opposite finger and thumb, until you reach the pinkie. From there, massage the padded outer edge of the hand between your thumb and forefinger. Using your thumb and rotating in small circles, move down over and across your wrist and back up toward the pad at the base of the thumb and across the lower padded area. Then work into the unpadded area of the palm, targeted each unmassaged area until all the reflex points zones have been massaged.

Take a moment to repeat the breathing exercises and then repeat on the other hand.

Ear Method

You can either do one ear at a time or both ears at once, whichever is easiest and most effective for you.

Beginning with the ear lobe, roll the skin of the ear around between your thumb and forefinger, working from the bottom of the ear around to the top. Once you have worked around the lobe and shell of the ear, starting at the head and working back around to the head, work around the inside reflex point zones of the ear in the opposite direction, until all zones have been covered.

Chapter 8:
Hand Reflexology:
Specific Tips & Techniques

- Hand reflexology is good for public spaces, when you can't do a full reflex point workup on the feet.
- Try using stress-relieving zones on the hands during phone calls with irate customers or similar situations at work where you feel like you might get upset and say the wrong thing.
- Trying copying the reflex point zones onto your hand the first couple of times you try the method, in order to help you remember where and what the different zones are. Alternatively, make several copies of the chart without the labels and write the zones onto the blank charts. This will help you work your way up to being able to fill them

all in automatically without needing to refer to the chart.

- Soaking the hands in warm water before a session will not only help you relax, but will help you be able to massage the reflex points for longer without fatigue.

- Talcum powder and corn starch help the massage and keep sweat from creating friction on the skin, but it can also get messy. Keep a clean dry towel close at hand whenever you are doing a session, either alone or with a friend.

- The frequency of your reflexology sessions is up to you. You can do long sessions once a week or do smaller sessions on a daily basis. Trying doing mini sessions during stressful times of the day.

- If you need to keep at least one hand free, but still feel the need for the relief that reflexology can provide, put a ball on the table or desk and roll your hand over it to put pressure on the appropriate zones.

- Unless a zone only exists on one hand, you should work the reflex point on both hands. The exception to this is when the pain is located only on one side of the body. In other words, if your left shoulder hurts, only massage the zone for your left shoulder and not the right one.

Chapter 9:
Foot Reflexology: Specific
Tips & Techniques

- Whether you are self-practicing or performing the art of reflexology on a friend, make sure the feet are clean and dry before you begin.

- Socks can be worn during a reflexology session, in lieu of talcum powder.

- While you cannot target specific areas of the foot or particular reflex points, you can stimulate all points by walking along a pebbled walkway.

- Performing the reflexology techniques in the bath can be done even if you can't reach your foot and you need to use the ball method. Simply suspend the ball from the faucet with a piece of string, so that you can easily manipulate it around with your foot.

- If you can't reach your foot and you don't have a ball to use to massage the reflex points, you can also use the rounded edge of an object such as a chair for the outer points of the foot and any long object with a rounded end which helps you reach your foot without bending, such as the end of a broom handle.

- Another way to stimulate all the reflex points of the foot at the same time is to fill a dish pan with marbles and roll your feet around on them.

- For muscle pains, it might be beneficial to work the reflex points that correlate to nearby areas of the body. In other words, if you are experiencing pain in your shoulder, it might be helpful to also work the zones on the feet that relate to your neck and your arm.

Chapter 10:
Ear Reflexology:
Specific Tips & Techniques

- For the smallest reflex point areas of the ear, fit an eraser onto the sharp side of a straight pin with a ball head and use the ball to manipulate the area.
- If the area is not too small, you can use the eraser end of the pencil to massage over the reflex point.
- Clean the shell of the ear with a cotton swab dipped in rubbing alcohol before beginning a session of ear reflexology.
- Do not put talcum powder in the ear or use it on your fingers when manipulating the reflex point zones of the ear.

- Since the zones of the ear are so small and particular when compared to the hands and feet and cannot be seen, it might be best to use a partner to assist you. On the other hand, you might simply find it of benefit to use a holistic approach and just massage the entire ear, so that all zones are addressed.

Conclusion

Reflexology is not for everyone, but it can be a helpful tool for some. The practice takes only minutes a day, but the effects on mood and pain level can be significant. By maintaining focus and relaxation, and repeating a few simple movements, you can learn to work with your body to combat pain and depression.

DISCLAIMER AND/OR LEGAL NOTICES:
Every effort has been made to accurately represent this book and it's potential. Results vary with every individual, and your results may or may not be different from those depicted. No promises, guarantees or warranties, whether stated or implied, have been made that you will produce any specific result from this book. Your efforts are individual and unique, and may vary from those shown. Your success depends on your efforts, background and motivation.

The material in this publication is provided for educational and informational purposes only and is not intended as medical advice. The information contained in this book should not be used to diagnose or treat any illness, metabolic disorder, disease or health problem. Always consult your physician or health care provider before beginning any nutrition or exercise program. Use of the programs, advice, and information contained in this book is at the sole choice and risk of the reader.

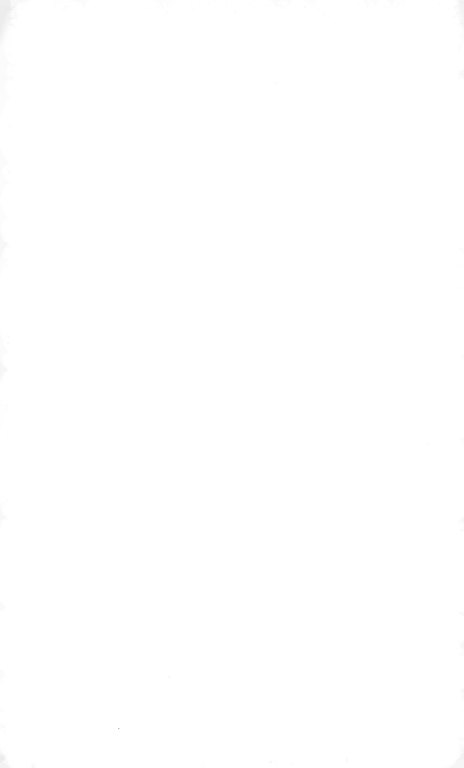

Made in the USA
San Bernardino, CA
12 September 2016